YOUR KNOWLEDGE HAS VALUE

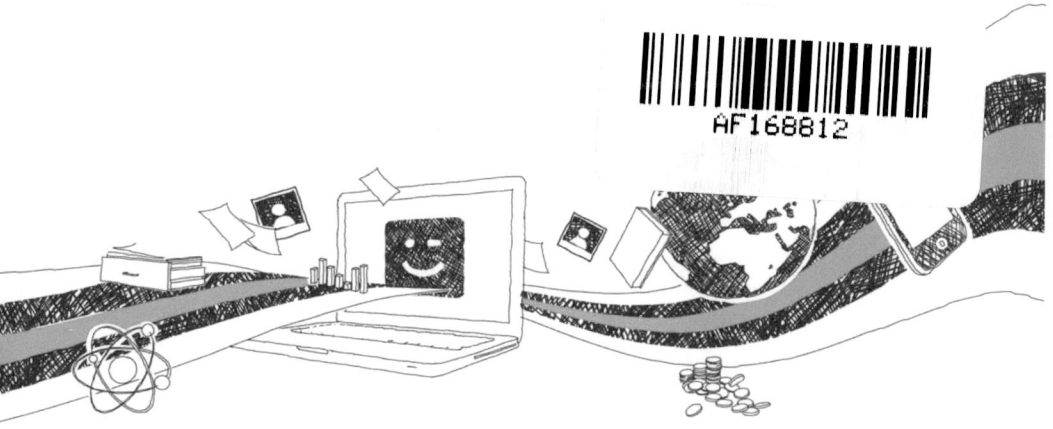

- We will publish your bachelor's and master's thesis, essays and papers

- Your own eBook and book - sold worldwide in all relevant shops

- Earn money with each sale

Upload your text at www.GRIN.com and publish for free

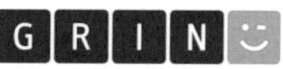

Bibliographic information published by the German National Library:

The German National Library lists this publication in the National Bibliography; detailed bibliographic data are available on the Internet at http://dnb.dnb.de .

This book is copyright material and must not be copied, reproduced, transferred, distributed, leased, licensed or publicly performed or used in any way except as specifically permitted in writing by the publishers, as allowed under the terms and conditions under which it was purchased or as strictly permitted by applicable copyright law. Any unauthorized distribution or use of this text may be a direct infringement of the author s and publisher s rights and those responsible may be liable in law accordingly.

Imprint:

Copyright © 2017 GRIN Verlag
Print and binding: Books on Demand GmbH, Norderstedt Germany
ISBN: 9783668971080

This book at GRIN:

https://www.grin.com/document/489776

Edikan Ukpong

Traditional Communication and Health Awareness in Abak-Akwa Ibom, Nigeria

GRIN Verlag

GRIN - Your knowledge has value

Since its foundation in 1998, GRIN has specialized in publishing academic texts by students, college teachers and other academics as e-book and printed book. The website www.grin.com is an ideal platform for presenting term papers, final papers, scientific essays, dissertations and specialist books.

Visit us on the internet:

http://www.grin.com/

http://www.facebook.com/grincom

http://www.twitter.com/grin_com

ABSTRACT

The study examines the uses and impact of traditional communication as effective tool for creating health awareness in Abak rural region. The study is predicated on the research problem that the Western modern mass media which have dominated the landscape of Abak rural region have not been very effective in mobilising the grassroots who are mostly rural, poor and illiterate for development. Adopting the survey research method using primary and secondary data sources a sample size of 175 drawn from Abak, were selected for the study. Simple percentages, tables, frequencies and charts were used to analyse the data. The findings shows that traditional communication is useful and effective for creating health awareness; traditional communication or media tools exist for creating health awareness; traditional communication media can be strategically used to reach the rural populace; there are significant hindrances to effective utilization of traditional communication media; and there are policies and projects that boost the use and impact of tradition communication. The recommendations are effective needs assessment, effective use of traditional communication media to reach the grassroots given their low literacy level, for adequate awareness, sensitisation and mobilisation for development, proper funding of traditional communication to preserve cultural values and heritage, greater involvement of traditional institutions and persons for effective creating health awareness.

Table of Contents

1 INTRODUCTION 3
   1.2 STATEMENT OF THE PROBLEM 4
   1.3 OBJECTIVES OF THE STUDY 4
   1.4 RESEARCH QUESTIONS 4
   1.5 SIGNIFICANCE OF THE STUDY 5
2 LITERATURE REVIEW 5
   2.1 WHAT IS TRADITIONAL COMMUNICATION AND ITS MEDIA 5
   2.2 TAXONOMY OF TRADITIONAL MEDIA SYSTEMS 6
   2.3 THE INTERACTIVE POWER OF LOCAL AND TRADITIONAL COMMUNICATION 8
   2.4 THEORETICAL FRAMEWORK 9
3. RESEARCH METHODOLOGY 10
4. DATA PRESENTATION AND ANALYSIS 10
   4.1 SUMMARY OF FINDINGS 12
5. CONCLUSION 13
6 RECOMMENDATIONS 13
REFERENCES 15

1 INTRODUCTION

Traditional media are communication channels which reflect the culture of a given group of people, most especially within Africa societies. These channels of communication are not merely introduced to the people like the mass media, but are part and parcel of the way of life of these groups of people (Nwabueze, 2007; Nwodu and Nwanmuo, 2006). Traditional media have also been identified as folk media or Ora media (Ugboajah, 1985) include the town crier, church, village square, market place, Igwe-in-council, dance or music, divination, native language, proverbs, folklores, etc. They make it possible for messages to be packaged and transferred in locally popular artistic forms. This cannot be rivalled by any other means of communication with regard to reaching the rural dwellers.

Also, traditional media refer to conservative means of communication as practiced by various global communities and cultures from ancient times. Folk media are some of the most vibrant representations of traditional media because they reflect communication channels for, by, and of the common people of a society or region. Traditional media are vehicles of communication which are rich in variety. They are readily available and economically viable. They win the confidence of rural masses, as they are still alive (Akpabio, 2011).

Traditional media are very useful to deal with sensitive issues of health, where face to face communication may not be suitable. During the freedom struggle, many of these performing arts have played a vital role in spreading the spirit of freedom movement. In our country, the government has been successful in spreading messages of family planning, polio immunisation etc. through traditional media (Wilson 1987). Therefore, communicators have to test different categories of traditional performances to identify the ones that are flexible enough to absorb development messages to meet the contemporary needs; flexibility is the most important factor (Udomisor, 2007).

However, today, it is a wide belief that the advent of New Communication Technology (NCT) has brought forth a set of opportunities and challenges for traditional media (Garrison, 1996) cited in Salman, Ibrahim, Yusof, Mustaffa and Mahbob (2011). The presence of new media, television, radio and then the Internet in particular, has posed a challenge to traditional media (Domingo & Heinonen, 2008). But, despite the pressure mounted on the traditional media by the new media, the place and relevance of traditional media of communication cannot be sidelined.

1.2 STATEMENT OF THE PROBLEM

It is believed that the mass media have dominated the political, socio-cultural and development space of Abak rural region. But they have not been all that effective in communicating and mobilising the grassroots who are mostly rural, poor and illiterate for development, politicking and other vital aspects that need the masses to force them into operation such as health. Consequently, there is a pervasive feeling of alienation and marginalization by the grassroots which portends grave danger to the people of Abak.

Thus, the traditional media which are rooted in the people's culture are considered very effective or more effective in grassroots mobilisation for development in health, in term of awareness and participation especially with the global paradigm shift to bottom-up approach to development and globalisation (which is contextualising global events to local situations). It is to this end that, the study which to answer the question: How can traditional communication be used as an effective tool for creating awareness about health issues and help the implementation of health policies to the rural populace of Abak?

1.3 OBJECTIVES OF THE STUDY

The objectives of this study were to:

i. determine if traditional media can be strategically used to reach the rural populace of Abak with health issues;
ii. find out how traditional communication can be used as an effective tool for creating awareness about health issues to the rural populace of Abak;
iii. identify traditional media tools used for creating awareness about health issues to the rural populace of Abak;
iv. ascertain the possible hindrances to effective utilisation of traditional media for creating awareness about health issues to the rural populace of Abak

1.4 RESEARCH QUESTIONS

The following research question guided the operation of this study:

i. To what extent can traditional media be strategically used to reach the rural populace of Abak with health issues?
ii. How traditional communication can be used as an effective tool for creating awareness about health issues to the rural populace of Abak?
iii. What are the traditional media tools used for creating awareness about health issues to the rural populace of Abak?

iv. What are the possible hindrances to effective utilisation of traditional media for creating awareness about health issues to the rural populace of Abak?

1.5 SIGNIFICANCE OF THE STUDY

The significance of the study cannot be overemphasised. It is so significant in the following ways:

It will enable the agencies concerned with creating awareness on health issues to known how powerful traditional communication can be as effective advertising tools. The study will enable the rural dwellers to compare and contrast between modern and traditional communication, the latter and more effective in brining development to their areas. It will also serve as reference materials for other the researchers and scholars carrying out research similar to the present study. In case, there are areas or issues that are perceived not to be treated in detail or comprehensively, the study will help to elicit curiosity, capable of inciting research interest in this area.

2 LITERATURE REVIEW

2.1 WHAT IS TRADITIONAL COMMUNICATION AND ITS MEDIA

Traditional Communication Systems refer to all organised processes of production and exchange of information managed by rural communities. Their tools, like traditional theatre, masks and puppets performances, tales, proverbs, riddles and songs, should be seen as cultural and endogenous response to different community needs for information, education, social protest and entertainment. These systems are often used to solve the contradiction between the need for change (development) of a rural community and the need to preserve its cultural values. After all, these values ensure that the changes are acceptable by all social groups of the community. On the other hand, all communication processes based on media which are not created and managed by the rural community themselves, like radio, video and television, are not perceived as traditional oriented and are considered external to the rural community (Ilo, 2011).

The traditional system of communication is a continuous process of information dissemination, entertainment and education used in societies which have not been seriously dislocated by western culture or any other external influence as is the case in many parts of the world. The system even operates in urban centres which have accepted to manipulate western media system for the purpose of enhancing the socio-economic development of these areas. Thus some methods of communication which hitherto belonged to the traditional system no longer operate because social and economic activities have made it possible to create the contexts of them. For example, communication with fire as a means of attracting attention or notifying a neighbouring community of an event does not seem to have a place today in any of our societies except perhaps among the mountain tribes and among hunters and adventurers in some places.

2.2 TAXONOMY OF TRADITIONAL MEDIA SYSTEMS

It was in 1981 that Des Wilson working in the Cross River area of Nigeria approached the virgin land of traditional media taxonomy through a systematic study, classification, analysis and understanding of the various media processes and content within the traditional context. The Theatre Workshop experimentation recommended by experts in Botswana in 1979 and studies by Nwunell (1981) have also contributed to our knowledge of the traditional media system.

There are numerous traditional forms of communication in Nigeria's old Calabar province. These are the various forms which the fabled town crier employs in his different communication roles. They can be broadly divided into eleven classes, namely:

(i) Idiophones: These are self-sounding instruments or technical wares which produce sound without the addition or use of an intermediary medium. The sound or message emanates from the materials from which the instruments are made and they could be shaken, scratched, struck, pricked (pulled) or pressed with the feet. In this group we have the gong, woodlock, wooden drum, bell and rattle,

(ii) Membranophones: These are media on which sound is produced through the vibration of membranes. They include all varieties of skin or leather drum. These drums are beaten or struck with well-carved sticks. Among the various Nigerian groups, skin drums of various sizes and shapes abound. Perhaps the most popular, because it is the most exposed and intricate in its craftsmanship, is the Yoruba talking drum, locally called 'dundun'

(iii) Aerophones: These are media which produce sound as a result of the vibration of a column of air. They comprise media of the flute family, whistle reed pipes, horns and trumpets,

(iv) Symbolography: This simply means symbolic writing or representation. Communication takes place when an encoder uses graphic representations to convey a message which is understood within the context of a known social event and an accompanying verbal message. It is a descriptive representational device for conveying meaning.

(v) Signals: These are the physical embodiments of a message. Many ancient signals are still being used for modern communication today. For example, in Nigeria, there is hardly a broadcasting station which does not utilize drum signals to draw the attention of its listeners to the fact that they are about to begin transmission for the day, deliver their main news broadcast or announce time, close down or prepare for the broadcast of the local or national leader. Some of the signals include fire, gunshots, canon shots, drum (wooden or skin).

(vi) Signs: Marks which are meaningful, or objects or symbols used to represent something are signs. Sign language (i.e. a system of human communication by gestures) has been developed for the deaf. Signs are associated with specific denotative meanings while symbols usually carry along with them connotative meanings as well.

(vii) Objectifies: Media presented in concrete forms which may have significance for a specific society only or may be universal through their traditional association with specific contextual meanings. These include: kola nut, the young unopened bud of the palm frond, charcoal, White Pigeon or fowl, white egg, feather, cowries, mimosa, flowers, sculptures, pictures, drawing, the flag etc.

(viii) Colour schemes: This is the general conception and use of combination of colours in a design to convey some meanings. Colour uses the advantages of pictorial communication by combining the speed of its impact and freedom from linguistic boundaries to achieve instant and effective communication. Among the prominent colours used to communicate different meanings among the Cross River people are: red, white black, green, yellow, brown and turquoise.

(ix) Music: Itinerant musical entertainment groups sing satirical songs, praise songs, and generally criticize wrong doings of individuals in society. Names of those being satirized or praised may be mentioned or descriptions of their physical or personality attributes, where they live, or what they do may form part of such songs. Such groups as itembe, kokoma, ekpo, ekong and age grade choral groups perform these functions. They are potent sources of information and the latest gossip. This is as Jacobson (1969:334) points out 'an unconsummated symbol which evokes connotation and various articulation, yet is not really defined'.

(x) Extra-mundane communication: This is the mode of communication between the living and the dead, the supernatural or supreme being. This is usually done through incantation, spiritual chants, ritual, prayers, sacrifice, invocation, séance, trance, hysterics or liberation. This is a multi-dimensional communication transaction which has become more pervasive in all societies most especially in Africa.

(xi) Symbolic displays: These would be cultural-specific or may have universal significance and some of their characteristics are shared even with primates e.g. smiling, sticking out the tongue, expression of anger, disgust, happiness, and fear, the way we walk, or sit, gestures we use, voice qualities and other facial expressions.

2.3 THE INTERACTIVE POWER OF LOCAL AND TRADITIONAL COMMUNICATION
METHODS

Traditional means of communication are very rarely taken into consideration by extension agents and technical staff of development organisations. They often ignore the communication process of a particular ethnic group or rural community: how the group produces and gets information; what media and tools are utilized; and what role do the "traditional communicators" play. They oversee the communication network and the exchange channels of technical and non-technical information within and outside the community.

Unfortunately, the interactive and participatory quality of many traditional communication tools and media is rarely mentioned. Many health communication specialists and extension workers think that the simple use of local and traditional media automatically guarantee people's participation and the creation of a good communication channel with rural people. The problem is not "which one" of the many communication tools available should be utilised, but rather "how" the media selected should be used. In fact, a critical analysis of the history of cross-cultural contacts shows that African communication systems have been used in the past by Christian missionaries, Muslim mullahs, colonial rulers and development workers to get messages across and to influence and change rural people's behaviour.

The process of interaction within the traditional media remained a top-down activity controlled by heath extension workers with only token participation from the villagers. While the field workers were responsive to inputs from villagers to problem identification, the way in which the problems were addressed continued to reflect their role as brokers of technical services and information. Popular theatre had not transformed neither their field work nor their attitudes and thinking ... (Kidd 1982)". This kind of approach, in itself, is not always useless, but it is very limited. For instance, "extension theatre" can give good results in facilitating a first contact between a health awareness campaigns and the rural community.

In contrast to the above approach to using traditional media, by allowing the rural dwellers to participate in the communication experience, with villagers themselves showed their own perspectives of their problems. Health awareness campaign in Nigeria world be more effective to encourage farmers, especially women, to re-adopt and to improve an old but helpful health method, take up new health pieces of advice and practices, etc. In each village the problem identification stage was followed by a discussion and supported by role-playing of how problems might be solved. An analysis of the underlying causes of the problems developed. This process helped to write a script for a local theatre village group to present their own play on the health issues discussed.

2.4   THEORETICAL FRAMEWORK

The Cultural Indicator theory is adopted for this study. The cultural theory states that, culture is a sum total way of life of a particular group of people. According to Barran (1999), culture is the learned behaviour of members of a given social group. Thus, tradition mode of communication is viewed as a part of culture. Besides, there are certain things in culture that show or indicate how people respond to messages. Such things are languages, symbols, of dressing and among others.

In this process, traditional communication carries messages that inform the people with cultural indicators and appeal to the people. Culture and communication are two items, which are closely related. The aim of any communication is mostly to inform the people and to change behaviour and attitude of the people on important issues such as health or related programmes. Most often, the objectives is difficult to achieve because planners of health programmes do not take into account the cultural circumstance of the target audience.

Therefore, a good knowledge of the people's culture is necessary if the campaign to achieve rural care delivery should be possible and the main emphasis of the use of traditional communication for enlightening the rural people, and educating them in the health programmes of the government. Equally, if we are to predict the behavioural attitude of the people towards accepting or rejecting the health programmes. According to Bell (1984), recognition and knowledge of the nature of culture is basic to understanding human behaviour. Knowledge of a group, a personal belongs, enables us to forecast his behaviour in any specific situation. It ramous the mystery which surrounds the behaviour of people from other culture groups. Thus, culture is a very strong influence on the implementation of any health programme involving people from different or the same culture background.

3. RESEARCH METHODOLOGY

This study adopted the survey research method using primary and secondary data sources. The primary data used for the analysis were data collate from a sample size of 200 respondents from the rural populace of Abak was selected for the study. Simple percentages, tables, frequencies and charts were used to analyze the data.

4. DATA PRESENTATION AND ANALYSIS

The data used for this analysis were collected from the self administered questionnaire. Out of the 200 copies of the questionnaire distributed, 175 copies were duly returned and considered valid for the analysis. The data were analysed and presented as follows:

Table 1   **Respondents Knowledge of Traditional Media**

Response	Frequency	Percentage
Yes	175	100.0
No	0	0.0
Not Sure	0	0.0

Table 1 above shows that all the sampled respondents (100%) noted that they know what traditional media is; hence the appropriateness of their participation in the study.

Table 2   **Awareness of Traditional Media in Abak Rural Populace**

Response	Frequency	Percentage
Yes	175	100
No	0	0.0
Not Sure	0	0.0

Table 2 present that All the respondents (100%) noted that they are aware the usage of traditional media in the rural region of Abak.

Table 3   Traditional Media Usage in Abak Rural Region

Response	Frequency	Percentage
Yes	139	79.4
No	10	5.7
Not Sure	26	14.9

Table 3 above shows that majority of the respondents (79.4%) said that the traditional media available in the rural region of Abak can be used as a medium for creating awareness of health issues. This indicates that the variously listed traditional media (in table 4 above) can be used to create awareness of health issues.

Table 4   Effectiveness of Traditional Media in Creating Health Awareness

Response	Frequency	Percentage
Very Effective	93	66.9
Effective	31	22.3
Not Effective	15	10.8

The table 4 of this work reveals that out of the 139 respondents that noted that traditional media in Abak can be used for creating awareness; most of the respondents (66.9%) noted that its use can be very effective while 22.3% of the respondents said it can be effective. From this, the respondents are of the opinion that the use of traditional media in Abak is effective in creating health awareness.

Table 5   Uses of Traditional Media in creating Health Awareness

Response	Frequency	Percentage
Yes	152	86.9
No	0	0.0
Not Sure	23	13.1

Table 5 shows that 152 respondents (86.9%) noted that traditional media can be used in creating awareness on health issues. Hence, the sampled group affirms that traditional media can be tool in health campaign in rural regions in Abak.

Table 6   Extent to which Media is used in creating awareness

Response	Frequency	Percentage
Very Great Extent	45	29.6
Great Extent	95	62.5
Little Extent	12	7.9

Table 6 shows that only 7.9% of the respondents said that traditional media communication can be used for grassroots development in the South East to a little extent. This shows that the respondents generally believe that traditional media communication can be used for grassroots development and health awareness in the Abak rural region.

Table 7   availability of hindrance to the use of traditional media for health communication

Response	Frequency	Percentage
Yes	115	65.7
No	50	28.6
Not Sure	10	5.7

Table 7 shows that there are noticeable hindrances to the use of traditional communication for health communication, some of these hindrances might be distortion of message, untrusted sources, time old message delivery, etc.

4.1   SUMMARY OF FINDINGS

The findings of this study revealed that in the rural populace of Abak;

i. Traditional Communication can be used for creating effective awareness on health issues and Abak rural dwellers are aware of these traditional media used for creating awareness of health issues;

ii. There are traditional communication media tools for creating awareness on health issues, which include town criers, folklore, small group meetings, town union meetings among others;

iii. Traditional communication media can be strategically used to reach the rural populace with health issues, with 93% of the respondents affirming the effectiveness of these tradomedia;

iv. There are significant hindrances to effective utilization of traditional communication media for creating awareness, such as distortion of messages, untrusted sources, etc.

5. CONCLUSION

Any message designed for the rural populace that does not share the same frame of reference with the majority of the masses that constitute the target audience before, and for whom the messages are meant, will surely not meet the objective of the project/program as such gesture will amount to exercise in futility. This is because most government and development agencies carry out their projects or programmes at the rural areas with the belief that they understand the villagers very well to be poor and therefore, have no choice, that whatever they (villagers) are given is acceptable by them.

Lack of education or improper sensitisation programmes hinder the full and better appreciation of most government and development agencies' plans/programmes/projects by the rural dwellers thereby making them ignorant, apathetic, hostile and prejudiced towards any development project that is destined for them. And, continuous preference and dominance of modern communication over traditional communication will adversely affect our traditional and cultural system, as this will gradually and surely erode our traditional values, norms and cultural heritage. Thus, for effective creating health awareness, traditional communication or trado-media is very critical.

6 RECOMMENDATIONS

This study recommends the following:

i. Messages and programmes/projects targeted at the rural populace should be well designed in line with the wishes and aspirations of the rural populace through adequate and thorough research on their needs.

ii. There should be adequate and proper education and sensitisation programmes aimed at bringing to make rural dwellers awareness the gains of health awareness, and this should be done through the best and most relevant traditional media

iii. There should be proper funding of traditional media of communication, as this will help to preserve our values, norms and heritage.

iv. There should be involvement of traditionally inclined persons (e.g members of a particular rural area a project is to be executed; chieftaincy Title Holders, rural-based youths and market women, rural-based clergy men/women, rural-based government/development officers) so as to ensure and enhance easy relationship which can only be guaranteed through goodwill, better understanding and co-operation.

v. In as much as modern communication promises and assures easy and faster mobilisation and development, there should be more emphasis on traditional communication than modern communication in times of rural project execution, mobilisation, support and development, this is because of the fact that the rural populace have been exposed to it and are so used for it.

vi. Again, the traditional communication creates a better forum for clarification over certain issues that might seem ambiguous, and this helps to guarantee better understanding and appreciation.

vii. At best, an integration of traditional and modern (tradomodern) communication is strongly recommended.

REFERENCES

Nwabueze, C. (2006), "Synergizing the Traditional and Modem Mass Media for Sustainable Development Communication in Africa" in Nwosu, I. E. and Nsude, I. (eds) Trado-Modern Communication Systems: Interfaces and Dimensions, Enugu: Immaculate Publications Limited.

Nwabueze, C. D. (2007), "Role of the Traditional Media in Grassroots Mobilization and Poverty Reduction for sustainable Human Development" in Nwosu I. E., Fab

Nwuneli, E.O. (1981), "Formal and Informal Channels for Communication in Two African Villages" unpublished paper presented to the Division of Communication Policies and Free-Flow of Information, UNESCO, Paris.

Ojobor, I. J. (2007), "Communication, Behaviour Change and Sustainable Human Development," in Nwosu, I. E., Fab –Ukozor, N. T. and Nwodu, L. C. (eds) Communication for Sustainable Human Development, Enugu: African Council for Communication Education, ACCE.

Okunna, C. S. (2002), Teaching Mass Communication: A Multi-Dimensional Approach, Enugu: new Generation Books.

Onabanjo, O. (1995), The Impact of Radio and Television Rural Development Programmes, Ibadan: Ibadan University Press.

Udomisor, I. W. (2007), "Communication, Agriculture and Rural Development", The Nigerian Journal of Communications, Vol. 5, No. 1: 175-190.

Wilson, D. (1987): "Traditional Systems of Communication in Modern African Development: An Analytical View point", African medical Review; Vol. 1, No. 2.

YOUR KNOWLEDGE HAS VALUE

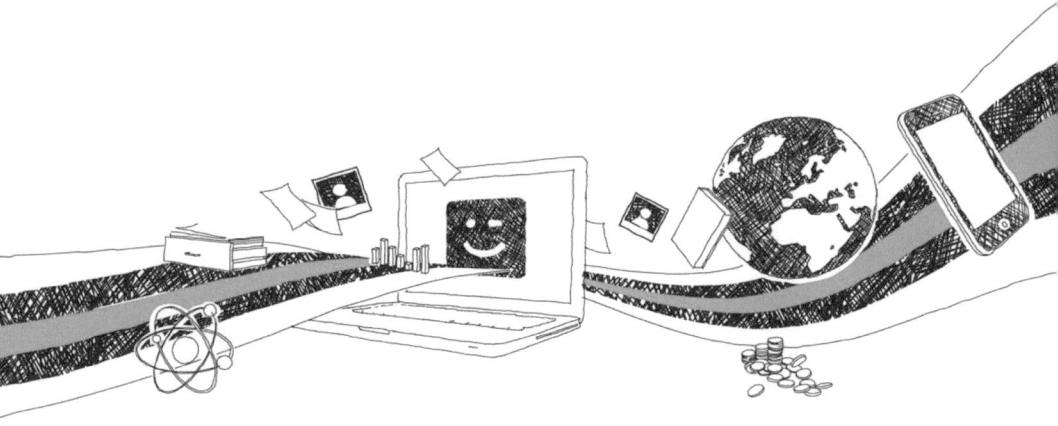

- We will publish your bachelor's and master's thesis, essays and papers

- Your own eBook and book - sold worldwide in all relevant shops

- Earn money with each sale

Upload your text at www.GRIN.com
and publish for free

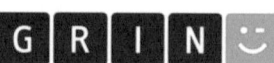